Sleep Solution

*Amazing Ways How to Solve
Sleep Problems Today!*

Table of Contents

Introduction

Congratulations on purchasing your personal copy of *Sleep Solution: Pave the Way for a Better Night's Sleep.* Thank you so much for doing so.

Are you sick of waking up exhausted and feeling famished throughout the course of your day? Do you spend most of the wee hours of the morning staring into the darkness instead of cruisin' to a snoozin'? Do you feel like you are missing out on certain aspects of life because you seem to be living amongst a constant fogginess? If some of these questions apply to you, I am here to tell you that it is time to stop the nonsense of not receiving the quality sleep that you deserve to get every evening. A lack of sleep can be detrimental to your overall physical, mental, and emotional well-being. No one deserves to live under sleeplessness' spell.

The contents of this book include:

- *The reasons why we have become terrible sleepers in general*

- *The science behind the process and functioning of sleep*

- *Simple things anyone can start to incorporate into their everyday lives **today** that will contribute to a better night's rest*

- *Alternative and natural treatments and methods to gather quality zzz's*

- *Utilization of methods such as meditation to help you sleep more soundly*

- *And more!*

It is time to stop living in the very unclear fog of sleeplessness and embrace life fully recharged and ready to conquer the challenges life has to offer. With a good night's sleep, those that are otherwise lacking in this area will begin to feel like brand new people. Learning independent ways to get a better night's sleep is an invigorating feeling! Especially since none of the ways in this book have anything to do with prescription or over-the-counter medications that may cause for more irritability, discomfort, and ruining your natural sleep cycle. Being able to take charge and tell the darkness, "Adios" as you float into the next day is something that will not only help improve the overall quality of the life you are aimlessly living but it will also aid in a longer life.

If you are ready to feel recharged instead of a fresh piece of road kill, you owe it to yourself to soak in the contents of this book. There is bound to be something to help you within its pages! Good luck my sleepy friends!

The following chapters will discuss what we spend over half of our lives doing - sleeping. While sleeping is an activity we perform every day, there are thousands of people out there who are not getting the quality of sleep they should be in order to function properly. It is time to put a stop to these endless nights of staring at your ceiling and time to put yourself to sleep!

You will discover how important sleep is to adequately thrive and survive and why we have more trouble sleeping today more than ever before. This book is packed with techniques, tips, tricks, and methods that can help anyone who reads it get a good night of rest. There are so many of us out there attempting to live life functioning on only a small time of rest or low-quality sleep. If you have gone a day or two without rest, you know how miserable it is to not only keep your eyes open, but to simmer down once the day is done and you are able to lay down peacefully in your bed once again.

It is time to put a stop to the non-sleep cycle and catch quality zzz's!

There are plenty of books about sleeping and how to receive better quality when it comes to catching the zzz's we need to thrive. Thanks again for choosing this one! Every effort was made to ensure it is full of as much useful information as possible. Please enjoy!

The Reasons Why We Have Become Such Terrible Snoozers

Although every single human being is unique in their own way, we are very similar in the fact that we all love a good, restful night of sleep. It is a crucial part in us being able to thrive and survive like we do. Without sleep, we would all be zombies, losing our minds and becoming almost in-human. Sleep is as important as fueling your body with the right foods and getting enough exercise throughout the day. It is as vital as it is inevitable. We cannot live without water and we cannot live without sleep.

Lack of sleep on a regular basis is a very serious medical risk that very few people take to heart. If a good night of rest is something that you tend to sacrifice a lot, make sure you read the contents of this book in detail. You do not realize how much you are sabotaging yourself when you do not allow your body to get enough sleep. You are harming your health as well as ruining your potential performance the following day. Sleep deprivation has been directly linked to severe physical conditions such as type 2 diabetes, hypertension, heart disease, and obesity. The good news is that if you do begin to achieve a better quality of sleep, you could reverse some of these conditions.

That being said, why is it that more and more people today have such a hard time dozing off when it is time to lay down and go to bed? This chapter will dive into the reasons why and there are some surprising ones that many of us do not recognize as sleep inhibitors.

Reasons We Cannot Sleep

Overthinking

It is funny that we tend to obsess over details that ocurred during the day when our head hits the pillow and it is time to get some rest. Why is this? Because unlike when we are fully aware and alert, we do not have the capability to refocus what we are thinking nearly as well. We typically do not have much control over our brain and what it thinks when we are going in and out of the phases of sleep. During the beginning, light stages of sleep, we may think we are awake but we really aren't.

How to fix: When you are irritablely tossing and turning, you are only keeping yourself from getting to sleep. Instead, make your way through the darkness into another room of the house. It is like magic that in doing this, your anxious thoughts seem to vanish. Then, you can lie down and manage to get back into a slumber. This easy method is quite simple and has been researched as to its effectiveness. It actually helps you from associating your bed with anxious thoughts and feelings. It is recommended to set a bit of an earlier bed time so that you can problem solve. Write down concerns and possible solutions a couple hours before going to bed.

Sleeping In

We are all guilty of sleeping in occassionally, especially on the weekends when we are free from workplace responsibilities. But late nights that are followed by extra time in bed actually throws your body out of whack, causing your internal clock that is controlled by nerve cells in the brain to not properly control body temperature and apetite. This is why Monday is rough for so many individuals. They stay up all weekend way past their bedtime and they feel pretty zombie-like when the morning hours of Monday roll around.

How to fix: Even if you do decide to or accidentally sleep in late, try not to sleep for any longer than an additional hour. Instead, take an afternoon nap of no more than 30 minutes to make up for lost sleep.

Your Partner's Snoring/Bedtime Issues

Whether your loved one snores loudly, tosses and turns in their sleep, sleep walks, or just makes weird noises, these are all things that have the potential to keep us awake or wake us up out of a peaceful slumber.

How to fix: Nicely ask your partner to try to sleep on their side instead of upon their back. There are also FDA approved pillows for all sorts of sleeping ailments that you as a couple can try out to alleviate issues that you or they may have during sleep. If that is a no go, get yourself a pair of earplugs that are designated for night time.

Change in Hormones

Women especially have issues at times when it comes to getting a good night's rest because of the major fluctuations of estrogen and progesterone right before and while they are on their periods. These changes in hormones can also occur during pregnancy and perimenopause. In fact, many women report that they will experience lack of sleep or troubles staying asleep way before they begin to have other symptoms of menopause, such as hot flashes.

How to fix: A couple of hours before bedtime, endulge yourself in a hot bath and pop a couple of over the counter pain relievers.

This is typically all women need to conquer their premenstrual symptoms. If your period is more stubborn, during the course of your period take a short-acting sleep medication. Make sure that you exercise 20-30 minutes a day if you can, especially if your body is going through perimenopause. This along with avoiding alcohol and major amounts of caffeine will assist in keeping you on a consistent sleep/wake schedule. For those pesky hot flashes and/or night sweating, sleep in a cool room and ensure your clothing is light. If you cannot get rid of the tossing and turning, maybe it's time to consider hormone therapy. It is safe for women over 50 that utilize it for no more than 5 years at a time.

You Are Hungry

When you head to bed hungry, those stomach pangs tend to keep you up and keeping your mind dwelling on the idea of food. This is why individuals who are trying to lose weight wake up so often hungry during the night.

How to fix: For a bedtime snack, consider high in protein options like a hard-boiled egg or a small serving of cheese. Protein will stick in your system longer, keeping hunger at bay while you snooze.

Your Sleeping Environment is Messy

If you are one that keep piles of paperwork, books, writing utensils, cups, plates and other unecessary things that really shouldn't be in the bedroom or wherever you sleep, then you are creating stress to yourself that you may not be aware of. Having a cluttered environment to snooze in actually plays a part in cluttering your mind.

How to fix: Keep a basket or other container that you can toss your unfinished work, paperwork, and other things in to set in another room. When you eliminate everything that has nothing to do with your time to recooperate, then you are signaling your brain to associate your bed and your bedroom with intimacy and sleep. It is also best to keep your computer/laptop in another room or somewhere where it can be closed off during the evening hours. You will then not be tempted to look at it during the wee hours of the morning. This also goes for phone screens. Plan to unwind from technology at least 1-2 hours before your bedtime. When you lay down and stare at a bright monitor, it messes with your body's ability to produce the hormone melatonin, which is responsible for informing your body and mind that it is time to go to sleep.

Lights in Your Bedroom

Lights from alarm clocks, street lamps outdoors, DVD players, televisions. and other appliances that cast any type of glow in your sleeping space can keep you awake. The tiniest amounts of light have the potential to enter the retina of your eyes, even when they are closed. It send signals to your brain to stay away and messes up your internal clock.

How to fix: If there are any lights within your home that shine into your room, shut the door. If you have an alarm clock with lights, turn it away from you towards the wall and eliminate night lights whenever you can. Perhaps purchasing one of those good ole night masks can do the trick as well. For outside brightness, buy some blackout shades/curtains.

You Can Hear Everything Around You

There are many people that wake up to the sound of a pin dropping. So sounds from traffic, neighbors, televisions, etc. can keep them wide awake during night time hours when they are trying to catch some sleep. On the flip side, there are some that if it is too quiet, they cannot sleep either. This is namely for city dwellers who are used to the sounds of traffic and people roaming the streets.

How to fix: It is not necessarily sounds or lack of sound that keeps you awake, it is the inconsistency of the sounds that can be distructive to your snoozing. If you need extra noise, turn on an exhaust or ceiling fan. This can act like a type of white noise, which will be consistent enough to block out other sounds that might wake you. There are also white noise machines you can purchase as well, where you can pick a sound to fall asleep to while blocking out other disruptive noises.

You Share a Bed with Dust Mites

If you do not clean your house or bedroom or wash sheets on a regular basis, you could potentially be sleeping with 100,000 to 10 million microscopic dust mites. These little pests leave behind residue that can cause one to have severe allergies.

How to fix: To reduce the number or existence of allergens, dust, and vacuum on a regular basis and ensure you wash your sheets at least a couple times per month. Ideally, once a week is recommended. There are also linens you can purchase that are capable of blocking mites. If you have a mattress that is more than 10 years old, it might be time to think about replacing it as well. As a final step, if you are able to, crack your windows and doors. Increasing air flow in a room is one of the most effective and cheap ways to diminish dust mites, or at least cut down on them.

You Let Your Pet in your Room or Bed

We have all been there when it comes to our beloved pets: you hear them howling or pawing at the bedroom door so you let them in. They usually try to get in bed with you, even though you do not want them there. So you spend valuable sleep time keeping them off the bed but sadly eventually give up and let them sleep with you. This can be majorly disruptive to your sleep cycle and pets in the bed are a great cause that keep people awake at night.

How to fix: Put a crate near your bed and let your pet sleep in their own bed within the crate. Dogs typically just want a safe and protected space and to be near you. Felines, on the other hand? Learn to ignore them when they come scratching at the door. Keep your bedroom door shut and set out special night time toys that will keep them entertained. Cats are nocturnal creatures and have a much different sleep cycle than humans do. If they won't stay away from your door, try double-sided tape.

The Science Behind the ZZZ's We Need

As human beings, we spend a grand one-third of our lives snoozing and gathering rest. Sleep is vital in retaining facts and things learned throughout the day, muscle recovery, and recharging the body back to full speed to take on the next day at full capacity. Because sleep is such a vital part of the way we live and since it takes up a big chunk of our overall life, it is time to dive into the science of what occurs while you drift away to your own little wonderland.

Sleep was thought to be a passive activity that we performed in which both our brain and bodies were inactive before the 1950's. But with just a bit of old fashioned research, we came to know that during sleep, our brains are quite active and that the activities our minds are involved in while we snooze is actually a very important portion of the quality of life we receive. But the main question that has yet to be 100% answered yet to date is why do we sleep in the first place? This inquiry has been a puzzling one for scientists and researchers of all kinds. Many think that it gives our bodies a moment to recuperate from the day we lived through. But, with a dose of science, the reality is that energy saved by sleeping a full eight hours is only about as much as it takes to toast a piece of bread. Researchers believe that the main reason we must snooze is because the process of rest is essential in managing normal levels of cognitive ability and skills like flexible thinking, innovation, memory, and speed. Sleep has been scientifically proven to play one of the biggest roles in the proper development of our brains.

What Happens During Sleep Deprivation

To really know the effects of adequate sleep researchers had to experiment what would happen in those that lacked sleep. I am sure we have all managed to pull a one-nighter a time or two in our lives and I know I can recall how I felt the next day after receiving little to absolutely no rest: irritable, groggy, and in a type of brainy fog. Researchers have found that even one night without sleep can greatly reduce our ability to concentrate, pay attention, and retain information.

Without sufficient sleep, the portions of the brain that deal with our sense of time, planning, memory, and language are greatly affected and will eventually shut down. One study proved that being awake for 17 hours can lead to a drop in performance that is just as equal to a blood alcohol level of 0.05% which is equal to two glasses of wine. It has also been shown that those who are sleep deprived are not capable of responding to changes in situations as easily or efficiently and they have a hard time making rational decisions.

Living with sleep deprivation not only impacts the way you function at the cognitive level but it affects your physical and emotional health as well. Sleep apnea, a disorder defined by an excessive sleepiness during daytime hours, has been directly connected to health problems such as high blood pressure and stress. Research has also proven obesity to be a side effect of not getting sufficient rest, because the hormones that control appetite are unable to regulate within our bodies normally since during the time we sleep is when they are released into our systems.

The longest recorded time for a human being to go without any sleep was 11 days which was done by Randy Gardner back in 1965. Only a mere 4 days into the sleep study Gardner began to hallucinate, particularly about him being a famous football player. Once the 11 days rolled around, somehow Gardner was functioning well and could even beat the researchers at games like pinball. Scientists have proven that amounts of adrenaline eventually make their course throughout the body after a period of 4-5 days, keeping individuals who dare to not sleep in an amazingly high functioning state.

The Sleep Cycles

From the time you lay your head down to rest and wake up refreshed the next day, there are quite a few things that happen to fully recharge your body while you are resting. Sleep typically happens in recurring cycles of 90-110 minutes and is divided into the categories of Non-REM and REM sleep. REM stands for "rapid eye movement." Your brain first enters the phases of Non-REM sleep and then goes in the REM cycle. Each cycle repeats itself until the time in which you wake up, so it is typical to go through about five rounds of these cycles total in the time you sleep 7-8 hours.

Non-REM Sleep

Non-REM sleep is made up of four different phases. During these phases, the body aiding in building muscle and bone, mending the immune system, and regenerating tissues. This type of sleep happens during the early hours of the night.

- **Phase 1: Light sleep** – We are half awake and half asleep during the first phase of resting. The activity in our muscles sow down and twitching from different areas of the body may occur. You can easily be awakened in this phase of sleep.

- **Phase 2: True Sleep** – After about 10 minutes of light sleeping your body will go into the second phase of true sleep, which typically lasts around 20 or so minutes. Heart rate and breathing slows down. True sleep is typically the biggest part of our sleep in total.

- **Phases 3 and 4: Deep Sleep** – During the time we are engulfed fully into deep sleep, delta waves are created by our brains. Delta waves are known as high amplitude or low frequency waves. Our breathing and heart rates at this phase are at their lowest levels. Phase 4 is distinguished by limited muscle and breathing activity. If we are woken up during the time we are within deep sleep, we typically do not wake up right away. We are groggy and disoriented for a few minutes before we are fully able to awaken. Sleepwalking, night terrors, and bed-wetting happen during phase 4 of Non-REM sleep.

REM Sleep

During the course of REM sleep we typically have dreams or nightmares. It is known as REM sleep because of the movements our eyes and parts of our bodies make during this type of sleep. The first REM period starts around 70-90 minutes after we fall asleep. During a typical night of rest, 3-5 cycles of REM sleep occur. Even though we are asleep, our brains are pretty awake, even more so than when we are awake and alert during the day. Eyes are rapidly moving around and our blood pressure and breathing rates increase. Our bodies are technically paralyzed during this time and researchers claim that it is our body's mechanism from acting out during dreaming. Once REM sleep completes its turn, the entire cycle of sleep starts back to phase 1 of Non-REM sleep and repeats itself. REM sleep is responsible for learning and developing a healthy memory and cognitive function.

It is important to remember that compared to infants and children, adults have different durations of sleep cycles than younger people.

Bodily Sleep Controls

The proper regulation of sleep relies on two main processes: sleep drive and circadian rhythms.

- **Sleep drive** is much like our sex or hunger drives in the way our body craves rest. Throughout the course of your day, the desire to sleep builds and reaches the point of needing fulfilled when it is time for bed. But when it comes to comparing hunger and sleep, your body cannot physically force you to eat, even if you are starving. But no matter where you are, driving or at a meeting, sleep can overtake you and force you to rest because you are tired. When one gets to the point of exhaustion, your body is somehow able to grasp periods of micro-sleep, even when your eyes are wide open. Napping only a maximum of 20-30 minutes a day can greatly improve cognitive functions. But napping any more than this can be a cause to decrease your body's natural sleep drive.

- Our body's biological clock is responsible for controlling **circadian rhythms**. This clock responds to cues of light, which boosts the creation of melatonin at night and then switches itself back off when it senses any kind of light. This is why blind folks have issues sleeping, due to the lack of light detection, they are unable to respond properly to light cues.

How Much Sleep You Should Be Getting

Just like we are all unique in various ways, the same goes for sleep. Not everyone needs the exact same amount of sleep to function properly. Researchers have said that the time for human sleep varies anywhere from 5-11 hours of sleep with the typical average being around 7.75 hours. A healthy night of sleep is crucial for the ability for our brains to adequately adapt to input. Lack of sleep enables us to soak in everything we learned during the day and it inhibits our ability to remember things in the future. Scientists also strongly believe that sleep holds the power to wipe away waste from brain cells. Sleep is also a crucial activity that affects the entirety of the body. Symptoms of migraines, high blood pressure, seizures, depression, and anxiety increase dramatically with lack of sleep, which also greatly increases the likelihood to catch illnesses and develop infections. Sleep is also a key component of having a healthy metabolism. Just one evening of missed sleep can have the potential to develop pre-diabetes in even the healthiest of people. As you can see, there are many connections that are vital to our overall well-being and the way we rest.

Aim for a Better Night's Sleep *Tonight*

If you found and purchased this book out of desperation because of a lack of adequate sleep, then this chapter as well as the next few are for you! There are many methods that do not involve popping pills that can greatly impact the quality of sleep you receive. Within this chapter are loads of successful techniques and tips that you can incorporate and try out, some you can start as early as *tonight*. Everyone is different, so don't become too discouraged if a method works wonders for someone else and does nothing to help you. There is bound to be a few of these methods that will help you fall and stay asleep so you will feel refreshed and ready to conquer the day that lies ahead of you!

Scientifically Proven Ways to Fall Asleep Faster

Enjoy Dinner by Candlelight

The less blue light that your body is exposed to before heading to bed the better! Bright lights of all kinds can decrease the body's capability to properly create melatonin. Besides the usually bright light culprits like phones and televisions, fluorescent light and LED lights can affect melatonin production as well when it is time to relax and go to sleep. This is a perfect excuse for a romantic evening. Break out the candles and eat around them and shut out all the other lights.

4-7-8 Breathing Technique

This breathing method was created with the mind of those that may need a healthy dose of help in falling asleep. It has been proven that it can assist you in diving into a slumber in less than a minute once practiced. This is because deep breathing slows down the rate at which your heart beats, which releases more amounts of carbon dioxide into your lungs. Here is how to perform it!

1. Take the tip of your tongue, placing it against the ridge-like tissue just behind your upper set of teeth. You will keep your tongue held in this location throughout the entirety of the exercise.

2. Completely exhale, your mouth should make a "whooshing" sound.

3. Close your mouth and then inhale to the count of 4 through your nose in a quiet manner.

4. Hold that breath to the count of 7.

5. Then completely exhale through your mouth, creating that whooshing sound to the count of 8.

6. Repeat steps 1-5 three more times, making a total of 4 breaths.

Utilize the Scent of Lavender in Your Bedroom

Lavender not only smells great, but its aroma has the power to relax nerves throughout your body which help in lowering blood pressure and assists you to get into a relaxed state for great sleep. There have been many studies that have shown people who have breathed and smelled lavender oil for about 2 minutes in 10-minute periods before bedtime raised the amount of proper deep sleep and felt much more rested the next day. There are many people who respond greatly to scent therapy and many who successfully use aromas in different aspects of their lives say it helps clear the mind, especially when the brain becomes active right when our heads hit the pillow.

Engulf Your Face in Cold Water

Especially for those that become quite anxious, distressed, or irritable right before bedtime, it has been proven that dumping your face into a bowl of ice-water can really help. When you are awake, your nervous system must eventually be reset in order to calm down when it comes time to sleep. Dipping the entirety of your face in really cold water triggers the Mammalian Dive Reflex, an involuntary phenomenon that acts to lower heart rate and blood pressure. Once you dry off your face, you can lay down with a sense of relaxed relief that will help you to slip into a nice slumber.

Wear Socks in Bed

I personally hate the feeling of socks on my feet while in bed and especially hate when the covers get caught on my feet. I am sure I am not the only one! But Swiss researchers have studied that having warm feet and hands helped with the onset of rapid sleep. During the course of this study, its participants used a hot water bottle at their feet, which was shown to widen the blood vessels, and resulted in heat loss. It is all about moving blood flow from the core of your body to the other extremities that might not get as much heat throughout the night. This shift of blood flow also helps the body product melatonin.

Enjoy a Nice, Warm Shower Before Bedtime

Getting your body nice and warm with a refreshing hot shower before bed, particularly after a long day already is a great feeling. But it can also help you sleep! After showering, ensure you step into a room that is cooler, which results in a drastic drop in body temperature. Many studies can prove that performing this simple action of quickly decreasing temperature within the body helps your metabolism work faster while properly preparing your body for a time of rest. Try to shower each night around the same time, which will help you not only create a consistent bedtime routine but it will also promote great sleep.

Keep Your Room Cold

To keep your biological clock in check, you must do things that keep your inner body temperature balanced. During the midst of sleep, our body temperature drops a bit, which many sleep experts truly believe helps us to fall asleep in the first place. The recommended temperature for your bedroom should be somewhere between 60-67 degrees to create the best sleeping environment. Both cool air and darkness cues your body that it's time for bed and it will kick into gear to produce melatonin to aid in sleeping. Melatonin is also responsible in assisting in the cooling of the body. Our bodies typically reach their coldest points anywhere from 2-4 A.M.

Hide Your Clock

While we toss and turn, we inevitably take a peak at what time it is and tend to groan at how much valuable time we are wasting because we are not within a deep slumber. We then watch the minutes tick by. You owe it to yourself to hide your alarm clock. Constantly checking it only raises your stress levels which make it difficult to fall back asleep. If you watch the clock like a pot needing to boil, you will only cause yourself to worry about the fact that you are unable to fall asleep.

Get Up and Do Something for About 10 Minutes

If you are awakened at any point throughout the night and you cannot manage to fall back asleep within 10-15 minutes, do yourself a favor. Get yourself out of bed and perform any kind of activity that utilizes your hands and your head, such as puzzles or coloring. Wake up with the intention to go back to sleep. This means veer away from phones, televisions, and computers. The blue lights of the digital screens will only inhibit you from getting back to sleep because it abruptly stops the creation of melatonin in your system. Avoid situations that may connect your bed and bedroom with anything other than sleep. It is all about respecting the stimulus values in life. Even your bed has one of these values! Your bed and bedroom should be associated with only sleep and sex, so when you are within your bedroom environment your body recognizes that those are the only activities it should be conducting itself in. Getting yourself up out of bed is hard to do, but is important if you cannot manage to fall back asleep. If you spend more time in bed during the day than what you sleep in it at night, stop that habit. This cues your brain to make your bedroom and bed a space for watching television, scrolling through your phone, worrying, and thinking.

Force Yourself to Stay Awake

This is one of those times that some reverse psychology comes in handy. You can lessen the levels of anxiety you feel if you force yourself to stay awake with your eyes open. It may sound funny, but studies have proven that this helps people fall asleep quicker than just lying down and drifting, especially in insomniac patients. Sleep just happens to be one of those activities that the harder you work at trying to perform it, the harder it is to achieve it. This is why reverse psychology typically is one of the better solutions to solving insomnia or lack of sleep issues.

Kick Your Coffee Habit to the Curb

While coffee is a great assistant that helps you to become alert and take on the tasks that need to be completed throughout the day, it certainly is not your best friend when it comes to getting yourself to sleep to receive a good ole recharge. Caffeine shifts melatonin levels that are produced within the brain, which can inhibit us from falling asleep at night and makes you believe that you do not need as much sleep as you really should be getting. Ensure that you drink caffeine no less than 6 hours before bedtime.

Same with Alcohol

Even though alcohol makes us tired at some point in the evening, particularly when we are done drinking and already drunk, it is one of the worst things you can consume regarding getting a good night's rest. Even though there are hundreds of articles that say drinking wine helps you sleep, it is not totally true. There have been numerous studies conducted that prove that those who even drink just 1-2 alcoholic beverages before heading to bed have a much harder time drifting to sleep and staying asleep. In fact, alcohol greatly increases sleep illnesses such as insomnia and apnea.

Stop Sleeping with Awful People

Those who find themselves in marriages or in other relationships that they are not very happy in find that it is difficult to fall asleep, especially when they sleep in the same bed as the individuals who may not bring them happiness but turmoil. Ensure that you go to bed with those who give you contentment. It has been scientifically proven that couples who are happy outside the bedroom tend to sleep better together than with those who argue and are unhappy in their relationship. It has also been proven that those who slumber well together tend to be happier couples overall.

Create a Bedtime Routine

Habits play a huge role in the quality of our lives and bedtime is no different. Creating and sticking with a consistent bedtime routine makes a big impact on the ability to fall and stay asleep. This especially helps younger children. Start the routine at the same time every evening and they will begin to associate that specific routine with the fact that it is time for sleep. Adults should conduct themselves in the same fashion!

Blow Bubbles

I know, this one sounds absurd, but it works! It is not as weird as it sounds. Blowing bubbles uses a type of technique that is quite similar to that of deep breathing. Blowing bubbles is also a great activity that is fun, mindless, and helps clear the brain for night time.

Figuring Out What Works the Best for You

All the methods within this chapter are about finding the center of calm needed to be able to receive an adequate and proper night of sleep. Like I mentioned before, every person is unique and there are going to be techniques that work and do not work and those that work better than others. Two of the big tips I can give you is to stop drinking alcohol and caffeine before bed and stop scrolling through your Facebook news feed at least 2-3 hours before bedtime. Keep a journal of what works and doesn't work so well for you so that you can keep track and are better able to incorporate what does suite you in your daily routine.

The next chapter covers some more creative and holistic approaches to gaining a great night of catching zzz's!

Tricks for Better Night's Sleep

Here are a few cool little tricks that could help you immensely at getting the kind of night's sleep you need and deserve.

Take a Trip through Your Day

Taking the time when you lie in bed to rewind through the most mundane details you performed throughout the day helps in the clearing of worries and other anxious feelings from the brain. Recall everything from sounds you heard, sights you took in, and conversations you had. This method assists you in getting to the mental state that is calm and ready for Z-catching.

Roll Your Eyes

Not at your parents! When you lie down, close your tired eyes and roll your eyeballs. This stimulates what your eyes physically do when you fall into a deep slumber and can assist in triggering melatonin production to get you to sleep faster.

Holistic Approaches to Aid in the Sleeping Process

The methods in this chapter will not only help you to get a much better night of sleep but are great techniques to improve your overall quality of life in various aspects of your life. These methods are successfully used to conquer depression, erase anxious thoughts and feelings, and promote overall happiness.

Find Your Happy Place

The reason much of the population does not sleep very well is due to all those thoughts bouncing around rapidly around our minds when our heads hit the pillow. This can be frustrating, trust me, I know. This is where visualization techniques come into play in helping you drift to sleep. Visualization helps your brain refocus on something pleasant rather than all the stresses and worries that you can do nothing about anyway once you hit the hay. Visualization can provide you with a sense of calmness that is a necessity when falling asleep. You can utilize visualization techniques anywhere. They are typically used in those that need to find a safe place to calm their mind during a stressful time to relax themselves. Usually it is not used to help one fall asleep, but it can certainly be used just as effectively to calm the mind enough so that you are able to get some rest. Visualization becomes easier with practice. Here is one simple visualization technique you can use to help yourself fall into a slumber:

- **The blackboard technique** – This one is very simple in all you must visualize yourself doing is standing in front of a blackboard with an eraser. This technique works wonders because your mind becomes less attached to the thoughts, feelings, and ideas pestering it and keeping it from sleeping by keeping your closed eyes focused on the writing of numbers on the imagined blackboard. If you continuously practice the following steps every evening, your brain will become much stronger and can quickly fall asleep when conducting this exercise.

- Imagine a chalkboard that is as big as you and stand in front of it.

- Write the number 100 in chalk on the board as large as you can.

- Then visualize yourself erasing the number 100 from the board, ensuring that you are erasing as slow as possible.

- Write the number 99 on the board and perform the same erasing action.

- Continue to count down the numbers you write upon the board until you drift to sleep. Once you practice this enough, you may find yourself only having to count to 96 before falling into a nice, peaceful slumber.

Listen to Music

There have been numerous studies of various natures that prove the positive effects that music has on our life. Being able to catch the zzz's we need to thrive is no exception. Studies have shown that listening to classical music helps with relaxation and even improves the quality of sleep we receive. You do not necessarily have to listen to classical music, especially if you are like me with it not really being your style. Pick out songs that are calming in nature or that help you think happy, positive thoughts and listen to them for about 45 minutes before your bedtime. Listening to calming music has been directly linked to lower levels of anxiety and depression as well. It is truly a win-win!

Use Progressive Relaxation Techniques

This method of getting a good night's sleep has been proven and is highly recommended by the National Sleep Foundation. It involves the relaxation of the muscle groups within your body through the means of slowing tensing then up and then releasing the tension.

- Begin this exercise by tensing and relaxing the muscles within your feet and toes. Tense up your muscles for at least 5 seconds and then relax them for 30 seconds.

- Perform this simple tensing/relaxing activity throughout your body, working your way up to the muscles in your neck and head.

- You do not have to start at the feet, but can work your way from your head to your toes as well. Whichever works the best for you!

- Repeat going up and down your body as many times as you deem necessary for you to become relaxed enough to sleep.

Breathe through Your Left Nostril

This technique is one utilized in yoga that helps in the reduction of blood pressure levels.

- Lay down on your left side with your finger on your right nostril, closing it off from breathing in air. Begin to slowly breathe in with your left nostril. This is a technique that is highly recommended to women who experience hot flashes during menopause and prevents them from getting so overheated that it inhibits sleep.

Meditation

We have all been there: after a long day, we just want to unwind, relax, and recharge. But our brains have ironic way of not letting that happen, causing us to overthink when our heads hit the pillow. But meditation can be a way to shut that pondering switch off in the brain. With the practice of one of all the following mediation tactics, you will find that your quality of sleep may drastically improve.

- **Make yourself yawn** – Mimicking the action of yawning has been proven to help fall asleep faster. It turns on many feel-food feelings, including the release of tension in the delicate area of the mouth and neck. Even though it may feel weird to fake yawn, you are releasing loads of tension that the day's stresses piled upon you.

- **Visualize the breaths you take in color** – I know this one sounds a bit interesting, but it has been proven to work wonders. This visualization technique allows your brain to focus on creating colors instead of on outside noises and other distracting aspects that keep you from sleeping.

  - Imagine one color in your mind with your eyes closed as you breathe. For one example, inhale blue and exhale blue.

○ Then pause and move on to another color. Inhale purple and exhale purple. Pause between each color.

○ Repeat until you fall into a nice, restful sleep.

- **Mindful meditation** – This process involves homing in on the various aspects of your life before you go to sleep. This helps your brain earn the ability to rest and you are more capable of letting negative things go. Focus on one issue or thought at a time and mentally let it go. I like to personally imagine myself putting problems that I don't want to hold onto right into a big balloon. Then once I have gone through everything, I mentally let that balloon go and watch it float away. For others, it is recommended to write daily in a journal. Take the time to jot down things for 15-20 minutes before bedtime. This triggers your brain to realize that once the lights turn off and darkness takes over, there is nothing you can do right now about the things that might be poking fun at your mind and that you will be able to better solve them the next day with adequate rest.

- **Using Mantras** – Create a personal and positive phrase such as "I appreciate..." or "I am grateful for..." Repeat these mantras until your mind is clear and able to focus on a single phrase. Try to end with an extremely positive mantra. This will help put your mind at ease, aiding a great night's rest.

- **Hum to yourself** – Performing this humming exercise creates a calming sensation throughout your body. Sit comfortably, close your eyes, drop/relax your shoulder and jaw while keeping your mouth in a closed position.

Inhale through your nose as deeply as you comfortably can, making sure that your abdominal rises instead of your chest. Then exhale gently out of your mouth with your lips together so that you create a humming sound. Take notice how your chest vibrates as a result. Perform these actions 6-7 times and take a few moments to sit quietly. Keep telling yourself that you are ready to go to sleep as you slowly make your way to bed.

Aromatherapy

This method was slightly discussed in the last chapter with the use of breathing in lavender scents. Breathing in and utilizing essential oils such as chamomile, ylang ylang, and lavender (to name a few) can automatically calm your otherwise bustling mind. These do not only have to be taken in through your sense of smell. They can also be physically applied to trigger areas throughout the body.

- Drip a couple drops of your favorite calming oil onto your pillowcase and then onto your temples before going to bed.

- Massage the oil into your temples to wipe away tensions you picked up throughout the course of the day.

Abdominal Breathing

Paying attention to breathing from your abdomen can help in the process of becoming more relaxed to promote sleepiness. This technique can be utilized during bedtime and throughout the day as well. It is recommended to pair this deep breathing with activities such as listening to calming tunes, closing of the eyes, or lying within a dark room. Turn your focus to the breaths and the ways they come in and escape from your body. To help with refocusing your attention, place your hands on your stomach while you breathe lying down. Hone your mind in on the slight up and down movement of your hands. This will help take away the stresses of the day that have accumulated and distracts you to focus on something relaxing and calming, which aids in the ability to drift to sleep.

Guided Imagery

This is also a type of visualization and functions by imagining a calm scene. This can be used throughout the course of the day as well as it can be used as a type of method to get yourself to sleep. You can imagine anything, from beaches, clouds, oceans, mountains, etc. Anywhere that brings you a sense of peace and harmony is what you are aiming to imagine. Pick places that you feel safe for your mind to dwell in. Guided imagery can be done by yourself or with the help of a therapist of imagery videos that can be located in many places online.

Once you have a place that you would like to imagine yourself in, utilize all your scents to explore that scene. What does it smell, feel, look, or sound like? The more detail you put into your image, the better able you will fall asleep in a calmed state of mind. Once you have practiced guided imagery many times, it will be easy for you to visit your place of comfort.

Counting Down

As you lie in bed, stare upwards at your darkened ceiling. Eye strain is scientifically proven to relax you ironically.

- Take in a nice deep abdominal breath and hold it.

- When exhaling, let your entire body relax.

- Repeat the last 2 steps 1-2 more times.

- Imagine yourself throughout this process walking down some stairs or up a gently sloping hill as you're counting down from the number 20 with each number determining a movement up or downward. Exhale after each imaginary step you take.

Yoga Breathing

Also known as 'Pranayama' breathing, this is known as the "life force" regarding performing yoga. Take deep breaths in and exhale slowing through just your nostrils. Ensure that you allow for the air you take in to drag over the back of the throat so that an ocean-like sound occurs when you inhale and exhale. This is the warm up breathing exercise. Once you feel properly warmed up, switch to square breathing. You perform square breathing by inhaling to the count of 4, holding for 2, and exhaling to the count of 4. Repeat this for 2-3 minutes or until you feel very relaxed.

Find a Trigger

This trick makes the mind focus on a specific action as you lie in bed and start to drift to sleep. Do something like stroking your cheek as you start to nod off. Hone in on what the movement feels like on the area you are touching as well as what your fingertips feel like performing the action. If you use the same action on a nightly basis, your body will associate it with sleep, so when you are ever having issues falling asleep, you can physically convince your body to drift into a peaceful slumber.

Make a Worry List

Looking through a to-do list or pondering over the things you have still yet to accomplish, especially things that have deadlines, will only lead to excess stress that keeps you from sleeping. Before heading to bed, write down the things you are worried about or the things you know you need to get done. This way, your brain is triggered to realize that you cannot do anything about them in the moments before bedtime, but rather as items you can conquer tomorrow after becoming recharged once again.

Or instead of physically writing things down, imagine yourself putting mental notes away in a filing system in your mind. This will aid in a calmer and better quality of sleep.

Natural and Alternative Treatments for Quality Rest

Give Yourself Acupressure

Stemmed from the process of acupuncture, acupressure is a technique that is classified as an alternative medicine that involves bringing flows of energy to specific areas of the body. Pressing on specific points and giving them pressure allows your body to restore balance within these various areas throughout the entire body. It helps you to regulate the body, mind, and spirit. Chinese medical history has shown many success stories regarding this practice when it came to getting a better night of sleep as well.

- Begin between your eyebrows. There is a depression in that location, right above the nose. Gently apply pressure to that area for a total of 1 minute.

- Now find the depression between your first and second toes located on the top of the foot and press there for a few minutes until you feel a slightly dull ache.

- Look at your foot as if it is split up into 3 sections, starting at the tips of the toes and ending at your heel. Find the area that makes up the one-third of your foot that is behind the tips of the toes and press there for a few minutes.

- Now apply just enough pressure to make for a nice massage behind your ears and massage behind them for 1 minute.

Foods that Help You Sleep

There are various items you can consume throughout the day that can aid greatly in helping you gain the deep, recharging type of sleep you so desperately crave. All these items have within them natural remedies that aid and promote better quality of sleep.

- **Walnuts** – Walnuts contain a grand source of the sleep-enhancing amino acid tryptophan, which aids in the production of serotonin and melatonin. It has also been found that these nuts contain their own amounts of melatonin as well.

- **Almonds** – Almonds are rich with a mineral that is necessary to get a good quality of sleep, magnesium. There are many studies to prove the negative effects that a lack of magnesium within the body can have, one of them being the inability to stay asleep once drifting into slumber.

- **Cheese and Crackers** – There is an old tale that warm milk makes you sleepy. This is true, but dairy products overall aid in sleeping. Calcium, which is found in almost all these items, assists in the brain's utilization of tryptophan. Calcium is also responsible in the regulation of muscle movements.

- **Lettuce** – Having a healthy salad with your dinner can help in the speeding up of the bedtime process. Lettuce contains a sedative property known as lactucarium which affects the brain similarly to opium.

- **Pretzels** – Yummy items like corn chips and pretzels contain a high glycemic index. With their consumption comes a dramatic spike in blood sugars which results in shortened times it takes you to drift to sleep.

- **Tuna** – Salmon, halibut, and tuna are fish that contain high levels of vitamin B6, which you need for your body to properly make melatonin and serotonin. Other foods with B6 are pistachios and raw garlic.

- **Rice** – Rice not only helps you to feel full longer but is also high in the glycemic index, so it helps slash down the time it takes to fall asleep. Specifically, consuming jasmine rice has been proven to help its consumers get shut-eye much faster.

- **Cherry Juice** – Drinking a nice cold glass of cherry juice before bed helps with the natural boost of melatonin levels. There have been studies that improve quality of sleep in insomnia patients who started to regularly drink cherry juice 1-2 hours before bed. The more tart the flavor, the better!

- **Cereal** – A neat bowl of your favorite flakes can aid in sleep. This good bedtime snack has two things needed for great sleep: carbohydrates and calcium.

- **Chamomile Tea** – This kind of tea is known as a stress buster. Drinking a cup of chamomile tea before bed increases glycine, a bodily chemical that aids in nerve and muscle relaxation. It also acts like a type of mild sedative.

- **Passion Fruit Tea** – Drinking a cup of this tea at least 1 hour before bedtime helps those who consume it to sleep much more soundly throughout the nighttime. Harman alkaloid, a chemical that is found within the passion fruit flower, is said to make changes to your nervous system when consumed, resulting in making you tired.

- **Honey** – Known as a natural sugar, honey has many different benefits. Regarding getting better sleep, it raises insulin levels that let tryptophan enter the brain. Mix a teaspoon of honey with chamomile tea for a great, natural sleep aid.

- **Kale** – Leafy veggies like kale are full of calcium, which boosts our body's ability to utilize tryptophan that promotes the production of melatonin. Mustard greens and spinach are other great options!

- **Lobster and Shrimp** – Here is a great reason to indulge in your favorite seafoods! All kinds of crustaceans are loaded with sources of tryptophan, which can bring on much easier sleep.

- **Hummus** – Chickpeas, which are the main ingredients of hummus, are a great source of tryptophan. So, eat some hummus on delicious whole grain crackers as a good bedtime snack or before you indulge yourself in an afternoon catnap.

- **Elk**- This game meat has twice the amount of tryptophan than meats such as turkey, which means you have the potential to fall asleep not too long after consumption.

Create a Daily Routine that Helps with Sleeping

There are many things that we do throughout the day that we do without the knowledge that we might be inhibiting our abilities to sleep later in the day. This chapter is full of the little things you can do regarding your daily routine that you can change to get better quality sleep when you hit the hay after a long day.

Limit or Avoid Taking Naps

If you can help it, try to avoid taking naps as much as possible during the day. Sleeping during the day can greatly inhibit your ability to fall asleep when it is time to hit the hay. If you must have a nap, limit your time to no more than 20-30 minutes. If you sleep any more than this you may feel groggier than when you laid down to gather a small recharge in the first place.

Exercise During the Day

Exercise of all kinds is something that we should be doing every day or at least 120-150 minutes 3-4 times a week. It aids in an overall improvement of health and mainly aids in sleep by reducing the stress we tend to carry around. Try to exercise no later than 3 hours before bedtime, otherwise the adrenaline your body produces while exercising may actually inhibit you from falling asleep.

Watch What You Eat

Instead of a big meal of steak and potatoes before bedtime, consume a lighter meal instead. Heavier meals are much more difficult for our bodies to digest, and trust me; indigestion is not fun to experience when you are trying to go to sleep. You should not go to bed hungry either, for the hunger pangs you may experience will keep you awake as well. Eat a light snack right before bedtime, such as hummus, Greek yogurt, cheese, or bananas (to name a few) to aid in better sleepy time.

Prep Your Bedroom

The place in which you catch your zzz's should be 100% free of gadgets of all kinds. Turn off the television and remove items such as laptops and phones. These items will only keep your mind too active for sleep because you are tempted to look at notifications. Your bedroom (or wherever you rest) is meant to get adequate rest, not for working or scrolling through your social media.

The lower the temperature of your room while you sleep, the better. The recommended temperature is right at 65 degrees. This helps in keeping your body temperature at a low enough number to help you fall and stay asleep.

Weighted blankets are great in keeping pressure on your body that aids in the relaxation of the nervous system that promotes a nice, deep sleep. The best weight to aim for is a blanket that is 15-30 pounds. It will feel like you are receiving a big warm hug from a favorite person, which is quite calming.

The higher quality your bedding is the better sleep you are more likely going to receive. Get a mattress that is comfortable and supports your entire body. Even though mattresses can be expensive, trust me, it is very worth the investment. Your bed is where you spend a third of your life after all! Ensure that you make your bed up with comfortable sheets and pillows as well. There are many kinds of bedding on the market. The better quality that your overall bedding is, the better your chances are to fall and stay asleep faster.

Dim the lights! As you have previously read, even the smallest of lights can greatly impact your ability to fall and stay asleep. With the help of installing light dimmers and/or wearing an eye mask, you can block out pesky lights that you may have no control over, like street lamps.

Control Disruptive Noises

Sometimes, just shutting the bedroom door is not enough to adequately block out noises that may come from within your bedroom, commotion outside, or from your neighbors. There are machines that are available to purchase that utilize calming white noise or ocean sounds that do a great job at keeping distracting noises at bay. Do your best to not rely on your phone to play these sounds.

Wear comfortable earplugs that you should dedicate just for sleeping time. There are many different kinds that are made up of soothing materials that are also easy to clean.

Establish Bedtime and Wake Up Times

Begin your routine that you perform for bedtime at the same time each evening. This not only helps you maintain a regular and healthy sleep cycle but it enables your body to fall asleep faster and easier. This is the same for the time you wake up as well. Do your best on the weekends to not sleep in for more than an hour at the most. Creating good sleeping habits can make a world of difference in your overall health as well.

Read

Reading 30 minutes to an hour before bedtime or reading to fall asleep is a popular way that people can successfully shut off their brains to the day's events and engulf themselves in an entirely other world that they can think about before drifting into a deep slumber. Pick either a boring or entertaining book that helps you get rid your mind of worries and things you need to do the following day. For sleeping purposes, stay away from self-help, DIY, or other reading material that stimulates the mind.

Practice Stretching and Relaxation Techniques

You have already become privy to some of the relaxation methods previously in this book that are great ways to wind down before falling asleep. Performing yoga or gently stretching various areas of your body before you lie down helps immensely regarding being able to fall asleep.

Utilization of Journals

I personally keep two journals, one that I write my thoughts and to-do lists down in and one that I document the dreams that I recall and take interest in wanting to remember. Doodling and writing worrisome thoughts helps you to relieve your brain in having to keep all those negative thoughts trapped within it. Jotting down dreams can help you see a pattern if you need to know of one, and for me as a writer, it is like free creative material delivered to me via sleep that I can utilize in future pieces!

Wear Comfy Clothing

When heading to bed, ensure that you are wearing loose fitting clothing that has the capability to stay cool throughout the night. Or you could sleep naked! This is probably the most comfortable way to sleep, for you do not have to worry about your clothing making you uncomfortable in the middle of the night or making you too warm.

Conclusion

Thanks for making it through to the end of *Sleep Solution.*

I hope that the contents of this book not only were educational and highly informative, but were better able to provide you with the knowledge you need to truly know how to get a great night's rest. I hope that the chapters were adequately able to outline some solutions that you could start trying out today so that you can perhaps catch some better zzz's as soon as tonight!

The next step is to try some of the methods and tips within this book to see which ones work the best for you! No one is the same, especially when it comes to achieving a great night of sleep. There is no reason that you should put yourself through another exhausting day or live in monumental moments half out of it due to lack of rest. As you have read, there are simple solutions to the science of sleep and you can utilize them to your advantage starting *today*.

So, as you conclude this book I leave you with this: to obtain a better life and to find the motivation to push through the day, you must not only learn but establish within you the importance behind bedtime and what it means for your quality of life overall. We all know how good it feels to wake up, stretch, and go about our day, knowing that we are charged and ready to conquer the day's tasks. It is time that you put sleeplessness to rest and stop letting low quality sleep rule your life. It is time to find a sleep solution.

Finally, if you found this book useful in any way, a review on Amazon is always appreciated! Thank you and good luck in your bedtime adventures!

www.ingramcontent.com/pod-product-compliance
Lightning Source LLC
Chambersburg PA
CBHW071142280526
45787CB00003B/1377